The Fastest Keto Diet Cookbook

Easy and delicious Plant-Based Ketogenic Recipes to Create Your Daily Meals in Minutes

Karen Yosco

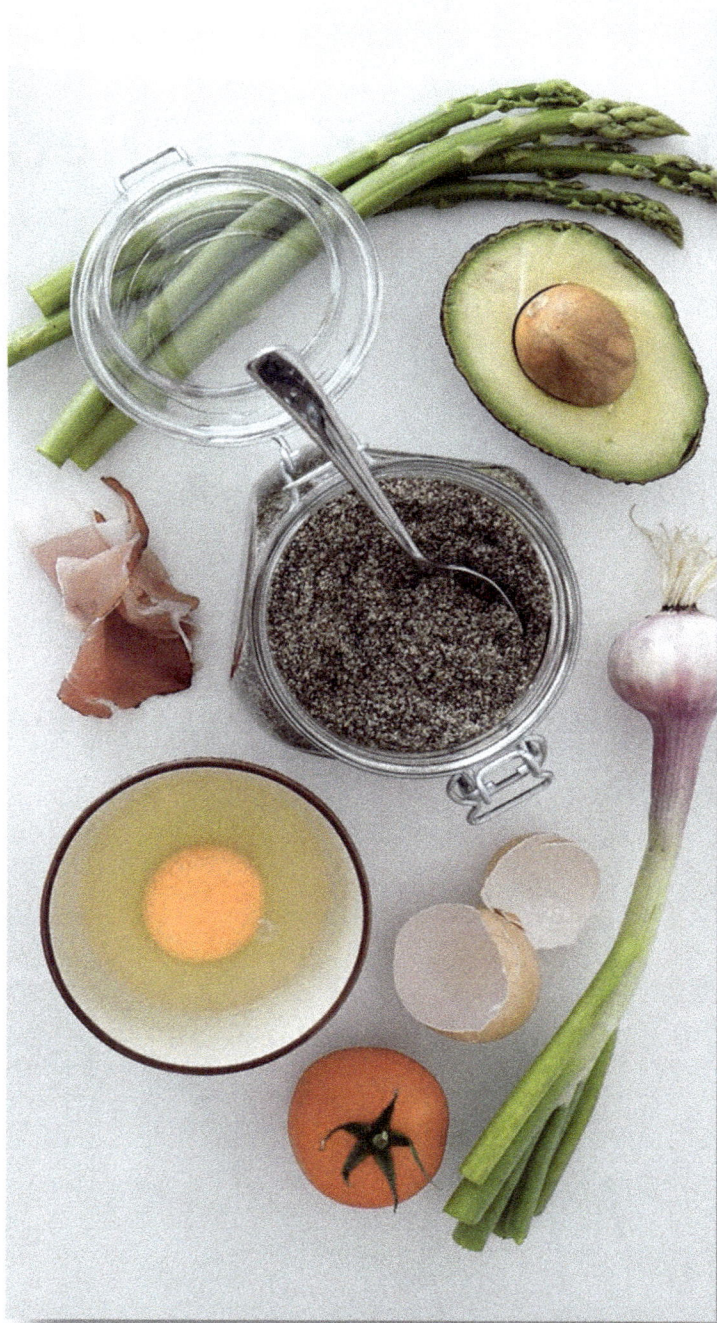

Table of Contents

BREAKFAST

Coffee Smoothie

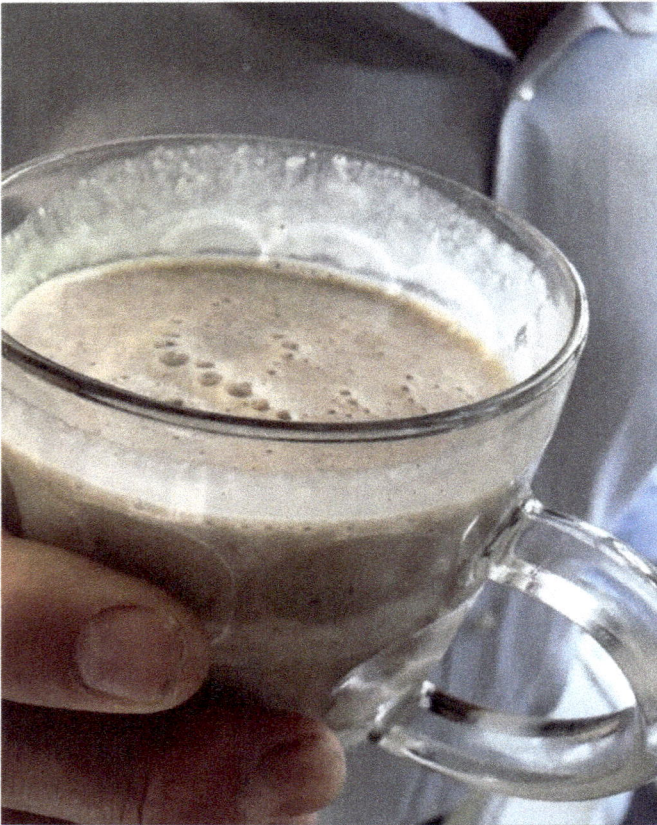

Preparation Time: 5 minutes

Cooking Time: 0 minutes

Servings: 4

Ingredients:

- 4 cups baby spinach
- 4 tablespoons hemp hearts
- 12 Medjool dates, pitted
- 4 tablespoons cashew butter
- 2 cup brewed coffee, chilled
- 6 cups of ice cubes

Directions:

1. Place pitted dates in a medium bowl, cover with hot water and let them soak for 15 minutes.

2. Drain the dates, add them into a food processor along with the remaining ingredients, and then pulse for 1 to 2 minutes until blended, scraping the sides of the container frequently.

3. Distribute the smoothie among glasses and then serve.

Nutrition: 391 Cal 15 g Fat 2 g Saturated Fat 60 g Carbohydrates 6 g Fiber 47 g Sugars 10 g Protein

Banana Cream Pie and Chia Pudding

Preparation Time: 1 hour and 10 minutes

Cooking Time: 0 minutes

Servings: 4

Ingredients:

- 2 bananas, peeled, mashed

- 2 bananas, peeled, chopped

- 1/2 cup chia seeds

- 2 teaspoons cinnamon

- 4 tablespoons coconut flakes

- 1 cup coconut milk, unsweetened

- 2 tablespoons maple syrup

- 1 cup almond milk, unsweetened

Directions:

1. Take a large bowl, add chia seeds and mashed bananas, add maple syrup and cinnamon, pour in almond and coconut milk and then whisk until well combined.

2. Cover the bowl with lid, and then place it in the refrigerator for a minimum of 1 hour until firm.

3. When ready to eat, distribute pudding evenly among 4 bowls, top with chopped banana, and sprinkle with coconut flakes and then serve.

Nutrition: 350 Cal 17 g Fat 4 g Saturated Fat 37 g Carbohydrates 12 g Fiber 19 g Sugars 5 g Protein

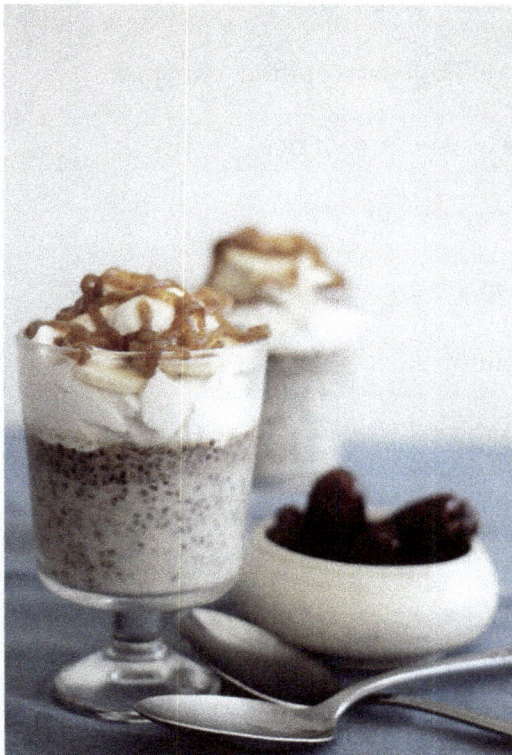

Brown Rice Breakfast Pudding

Preparation Time: 5 minutes

Cooking Time: 15 minutes

Servings: 4

Ingredients:

- 1 tart apple, cored, chopped

- 1 cup Medjool dates, pitted, chopped

- 3 cups cooked brown rice

- 1/8 teaspoon salt

- ¼ teaspoon ground cloves

- 1 cinnamon stick

- ¼ cup raisins

- ¼ cup slivered almonds, toasted

- 2 cups almond milk, unsweetened

Directions:

1. Take a medium saucepan, place it over medium-low heat, add rice, dates, cloves, and cinnamon, pour in milk, stir until mixed and cook for 12 minutes until thickened.

2. Then remove and discard cinnamon stick, add apple and raisins and then stir in salt.

3. Remove pan from heat, distribute pudding among four bowls and top with almonds.

4. Serve straight away.

Nutrition: 391 Cal 4.8 g Fat 0.6 g Saturated Fat 81.1 g Carbohydrates 5.7 g Fiber 24.8 g Sugars 6 g Protein

LUNCH

Rainbow Taco Boats

Preparation Time: 10 minutes

Cooking Time: 0 minutes

Servings: 4

Ingredients:

- 1 head romaine lettuce, destemmed

For the Filling:

- 1/2 cup alfalfa sprouts

- 1 medium avocado, peeled, pitted, cubed

- 1 cup shredded carrots

- 1 cup halved cherry tomatoes

- 3/4 cup sliced red cabbage

- 1/2 cup sprouted hummus dip

- 1 tablespoon hemp seeds

For the Sauce:

- 1 tablespoon maple syrup

- 1/3 cup tahini

- 1/8 teaspoon sea salt

- 2 tablespoons lemon juice

- 3 tablespoons water

Directions:

1. Prepare the sauce and for this, take a medium bowl, add all the ingredients in it and whisk until well combined.

2. Assemble the boats and for this, arrange lettuce leaves in twelve portions, top each with hummus, and the remaining ingredients for the filling.

3. Serve with prepared sauce.

Nutrition: 314 Cal 23.6 g Fat 4 g Saturated Fat 23.2 g Carbohydrates 9.3 g Fiber 6.2 g Sugars 8 g Protein

Eggplant Sandwich

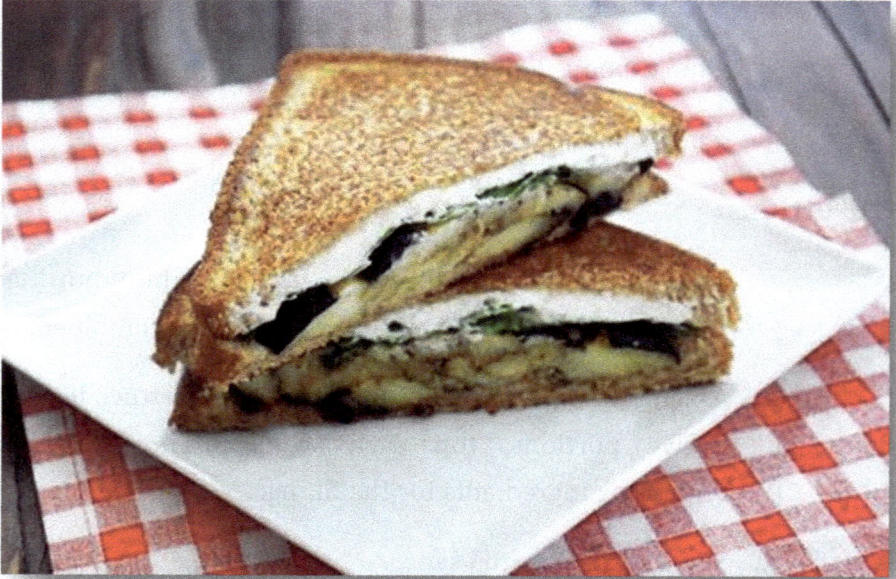

Preparation Time: 10 minutes

Cooking Time: 25 minutes

Servings: 4

Ingredients:

For the Sandwich:

- 2 ciabatta buns

- 1 medium eggplant, peeled, sliced, soaked in salted water

- 1 medium tomato, sliced

- 1/2 of a medium cucumber, sliced

- 1/2 cup arugula

- 4 tablespoons mayo

For the Marinade:

- 1 teaspoon agave syrup

- 1/4 teaspoon salt

- 1/4 teaspoon ground black pepper

- 1 teaspoon smoked paprika

- 1 tablespoon soy sauce

- 1 tablespoon olive oil

Directions:

1. Switch on the oven, then set it to 350 degrees F and let it preheat.

2. Prepare the marinade and for this, take a small bowl, place all the ingredients in it and whisk until combined.

3. Drain the eggplant slices, pat dry with a kitchen towel, and brush with prepared marinade, arrange them on a baking sheet and then bake for 20 minutes until done.

4. Assemble the sandwich and for this, slice the bread in half lengthwise, then spread mayonnaise in the bottom half of

the bun and top with baked eggplant slices, tomato, and cucumber slices, and sprinkle with salt and black pepper.

5. Top with arugula leaves, cover with the top half of the bun, and then cover with aluminum foil.

6. Preheat the grill over medium-high heat setting and when hot, place prepared sandwiches and grill for 3 to 5 minutes until toasted.

7. Cut each sandwich through the foil into half and serve.

Nutrition: 688 Cal 15 g Fat 2 g Saturated Fat 118 g Carbohydrates 7 g Fiber 7 g Sugars 21 g Protein

Lentil, Cauliflower and Grape Salad

Preparation Time: 10 minutes

Cooking Time: 25 minutes

Servings: 4

Ingredients:

- For the Cauliflower:

- 1 medium head of cauliflower, cut into florets

- 1/4 teaspoon sea salt

- 1 1/2 tablespoons curry powder

- 1 1/2 tablespoons melted coconut oil

For the Tahini Dressing:

- 2 tablespoons tahini

- 1/8 teaspoon salt

- 1.8 teaspoon ground black pepper

- 4 1/2 tablespoons green curry paste

- 1 tablespoon maple syrup

- 2 tablespoons lemon juice

- 2 tablespoons water

For the Salad:

- 1 cup cooked lentils

- 4 tablespoons chopped cilantro

- 1 cup red grapes, halved

- 6 cups mixed greens

Directions:

1. Switch on the oven, then set it to 400 degrees F and let it preheat.

2. Prepare the cauliflower and for this, take a medium bowl, place cauliflower florets in it, drizzle with oil, season with salt and curry powder, toss until mixed.

3. Take a baking sheet, line it with parchment sheet, spread cauliflower florets in it, and then bake for 25 minutes until tender and nicely golden brown.

4. Meanwhile, prepare the tahini dressing and for this, take a medium bowl, place all of its ingredients and whisk until combined, set aside until required.

5. Assemble the salad and for this, take a large salad bowl, add roasted cauliflower florets, lentils, grapes, and mixed greens, drizzle with prepared tahini dressing and toss until well combined.

6. Serve straight away.

Nutrition: 420 Cal 14 g Fat 5 g Saturated Fat 37.6 g Carbohydrates 9.8 g Fiber 12.8 g Sugars 10.8 g Protein;

DINNER

Chili Fennel

Preparation Time: 10 minutes

Cooking Time: 8 minutes

Servings: 4

Ingredients:

- 2 fennel bulbs, cut into quarters

- 3 tablespoons olive oil

- Salt and black pepper to the taste

- 1 garlic clove, minced

- 1 red chili pepper, chopped

- ¾ cup veggie stock

- Juice of ½ lemon

Directions:

1. Heat a pan that fits your Air Fryer with the oil over medium-high heat, add garlic and chili pepper, stir and cook for 2 minutes.

2. Add fennel, salt, pepper, stock, and lemon juice, toss to coat, introduce in your Air Fryer and cook at 350 ° F for at least 6 minutes.

3. Divide into plates and serve as a side dish.

Nutrition: Calories: 158 kcal Protein: 3.57 g Fat: 11.94 g Carbohydrates: 11.33 g

Collard Greens and Tomatoes

Preparation Time: 10 minutes

Cooking Time: 10 minutes

Servings: 9

Ingredients:

- 1 pound collard greens

- ¼ cup cherry tomatoes, halved

- 1 tablespoon apple cider vinegar

- 2 tablespoons veggie stock

- Salt and black pepper to the taste

Directions:

1. In a pan that fits the Air Fryer, combine tomatoes, collard greens, vinegar, stock, salt, and pepper, stir, introduce in your Air Fryer and cook at 320 ° F for 10 minutes.

2. Divide between plates and serve as a side dish.

Nutrition: Calories: 28 kcal Protein: 2.34 g Fat: 0.99 g Carbohydrates: 3.26 g

Bean and Carrot Spirals

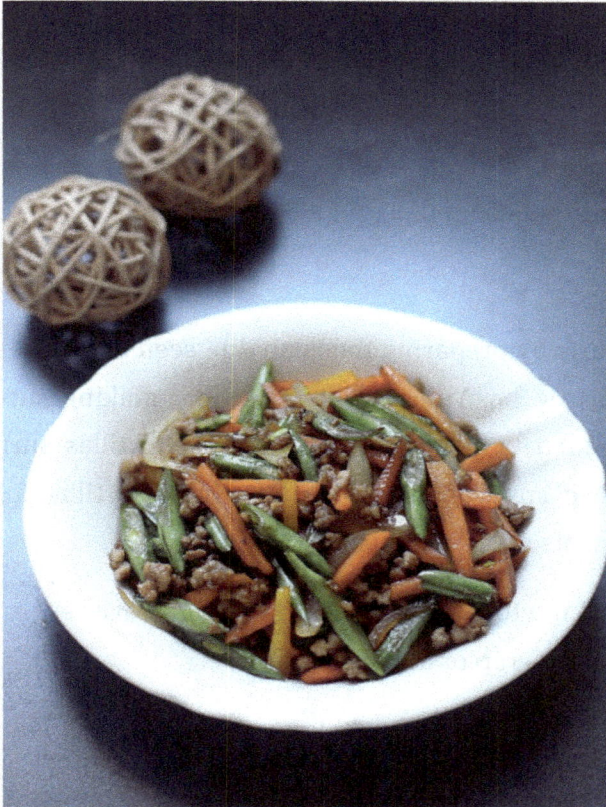

Preparation Time: 10 minutes

Cooking Time: 40 minutes

Servings: 24

Ingredients:

- 4 8-inch flour tortillas
- 1 ½ cups of Easy Mean White Bean dip
- 10 ounces spinach leaves
- ½ cup diced carrots
- ½ cup diced red peppers

Directions:

1. Starts by preparing the bean dip, seen above. Next, spread out the bean dip on each tortilla, making sure to leave about a ¾ inch white border on the tortillas' surface. Next, place spinach in the center of the tortilla, followed by carrots and red peppers.

2. Roll the tortillas into tight rolls, and cover every rolls with plastic wrap or aluminum foil.

3. Let them chill in the fridge for twenty-four hours.

4. Afterward, remove the wrap from the spirals and remove the very ends of the rolls. Slice the rolls into six individual spiral pieces, and arrange them on a platter for serving. Enjoy!

Nutrition: Calories: 205 kcal Protein: 6.41 g Fat: 4.16 g Carbohydrates: 35.13 g

Tofu Nuggets with Barbecue Glaze

Preparation Time: 10 minutes

Cooking Time: 25 minutes

Servings: 9

Ingredients:

- 32 ounces tofu

- 1 cup quick vegan barbecue sauce

Directions:

1. Set the oven to 425F.

2. Next, slice the tofu and blot the tofu with clean towels. Next, slice and dice the tofu and completely eliminate the water from the tofu material.

3. Stir the tofu with the vegan barbecue sauce, and place the tofu on a baking sheet.

4. Bake the tofu for fifteen minutes. Afterward, stir the tofu and bake the tofu for an additional ten minutes.

5. Enjoy!

Nutrition: Calories: 311 kcal Protein: 19.94 g Fat: 21.02 g Carbohydrates: 15.55 g

Vegetable and Chickpea Loaf

Preparation Time: 10 minutes

Cooking Time: 15 minutes

Servings: 4

Ingredients:

- 1 tsp. Salt

- .5 tsp. Dried sage

- 1 tsp. Dried savory

- 1 tbsp. Soy sauce

- .25 cup Parsley

- .5 cup Breadcrumbs

- .75 cup Oats

- .75 cup Chickpea flour

- 1.5 cup cooked chickpeas

- 2 Minced garlic cloves

- 1 Chopped yellow onion

- 1 Shredded carrot

- 1 Shredded white potato

Directions:

1. Set the oven to 350F. Take out a loaf pan and then grease it up.

2. Squeeze out the liquid from the potato and add to the food processor with the garlic, onion, and carrot.

3. Add the chickpeas and pulse to blend well. Add in the rest of the ingredients here, and when it is done, use your hands to form this into a loaf and add to the pan.

4. Place into the oven to bake for a bit until it is nice and firm. Let it cool down and then slice.

Nutrition: Calories: 351 kcal Protein: 16.86 g Fat: 6.51 g Carbohydrates: 64 g

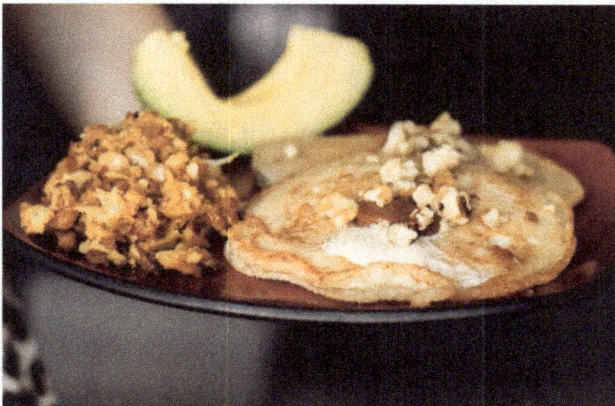

Thyme and Lemon Couscous

Preparation Time: 5 minutes

Cooking Time: 10 minutes

Servings: 6

Ingredients:

- .25 cup Chopped parsley

- 1.5 cup Couscous

- 2 tbsp. Chopped thyme

- Juice and zest of a lemon

- 2.75 cup Vegetable stock

Directions:

1. Take out a pot and add in the thyme, lemon juice, and vegetable stock. Stir in the couscous after it has gotten to a boil and then take off the heat.

2. Allow sitting covered until it can take in all of the liquid. Then fluff up with a form.

3. Stir in the parsley and lemon zest, then serve warm.

Nutrition: Calories: 922 kcal Protein: 2.7 g Fat: 101.04 g Carbohydrates: 10.02 g

Baked Okra and Tomato

Preparation Time: 10 minutes

Cooking Time: 75 minutes

Servings: 6

Ingredients:

- ½ cup lima beans, frozen

- 4 tomatoes, chopped

- 8 ounces okra, fresh and washed, stemmed, sliced into ½ inch thick slices

- 1 onion, sliced into rings

- ½ sweet pepper, seeded and sliced thin

- Pinch of crushed red pepper

- Salt to taste

Directions:

1. Preheat your oven to 350 degrees Fahrenheit

2. Cook lima beans in water accordingly and drain them, take a 2quart casserole tin

3. Add all listed ingredients to the dish and cover with foil, bake for 45 minutes

4. Uncover the dish, stir well and bake for 35 minutes more

5. Stir then serve, and enjoy!

Nutrition: Calories: 55 Fat: 0g Carbohydrates: 12g Protein: 3g

STIR-FRIED, GRILLED VEGETABLES

Broccoli & Brown Rice Satay

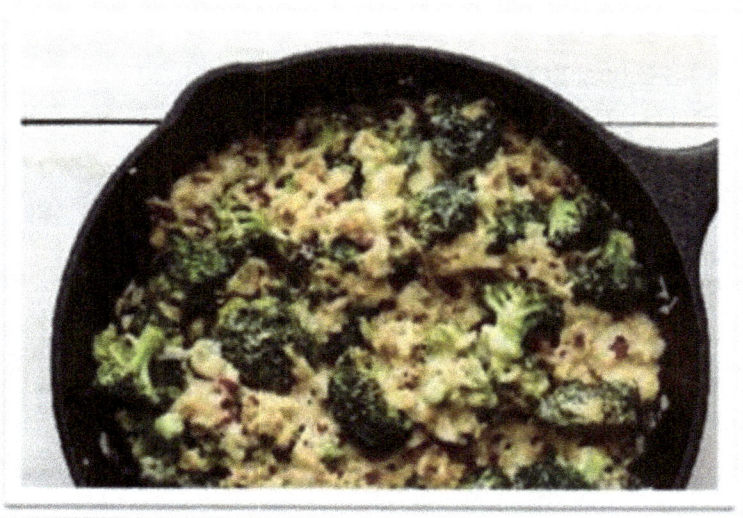

Preparation Time: 10 minutes

Cooking Time: 10 minutes

Servings: 4

Ingredients:

- 6 trimmed broccoli florets, halved
- 1-inch piece of ginger, shredded
- 2 garlic cloves, shredded
- 1 red onion, sliced
- 1 roasted red pepper, cut into cubes
- 2 teaspoons olive oil
- 1 teaspoon mild chili powder
- 1 tablespoon reduced salt soy sauce
- 1 tablespoon maple syrup
- 1 cup cooked brown rice

Directions:

1. Boil broccoli in water for 4 minutes then drain immediately.
2. In a pan add olive oil, ginger, onion, and garlic.
3. Stir fry for 2 minutes then add the rest of the ingredients.
4. Cook for 3 minutes then serve.

Nutrition: Calories: 196 Total Fat: 20g Carbs: 8g Net Carbs: 3g Fiber: 1g Protein: 3g

Sautéed Sesame Spinach

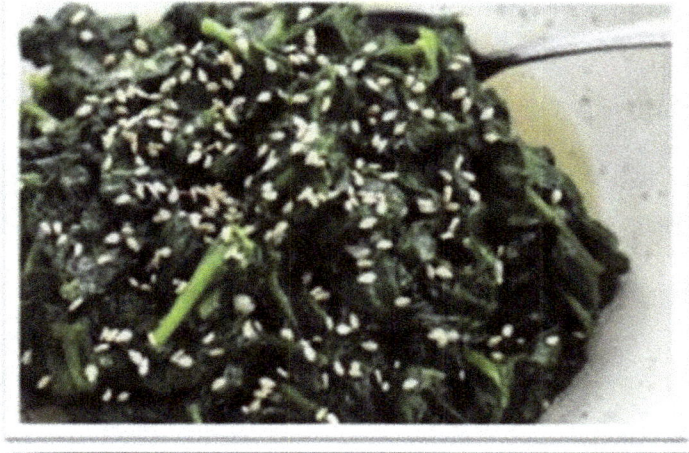

Preparation Time: 1 hr. 10 minutes

Cooking Time: 3 minutes

Servings: 04

Ingredients:

- 1 tablespoon toasted sesame oil

- ½ tablespoon soy sauce

- ½ teaspoon toasted sesame seeds, crushed

- ½ teaspoon rice vinegar

- ½ teaspoon golden caster sugar

- 1 garlic clove, grated

- 8 ounces spinach, stem ends trimmed

Directions:

1. Sauté spinach in a pan until it is wilted.

2. Whisk the sesame oil, garlic, sugar, vinegar, sesame seeds, soy sauce and black pepper together in a bowl.

3. Stir in spinach and mix well.

4. Cover and refrigerate for 1 hour.

5. Serve.

Nutrition: Calories: 677 Total Fat: 60g Carbs: 71g Net Carbs: 7g Fiber: 0g; Protein: 20g

DIP AND SPREAD RECIPES

Asparagus Spanakopita

Preparation Time: 25 minutes

Cooking Time: 25 minutes

Servings: 12

Ingredients:

- 2 cups cut fresh asparagus (1-inch pieces)

- 20 sheets phyllo dough, (14 inches x 9 inches)

- Nonstick cooking spray

- Refrigerated butter-flavored spray

- 2 cups torn fresh spinach

- 3 oz. crumbled feta cheese

- 2 tablespoon butter

- 1/4 cup all-purpose flour

- 1-1/2 cups coconut milk

- 3 tablespoon lemon juice

- 1 teaspoon dill weed

- 1 teaspoon dried thyme

- 1/4 teaspoon salt

Directions:

1. In a steamer basket, put the asparagus and place it on top of a saucepan with 1-inch of water, then boil. Put the cover and let it steam for 5 minutes or until it becomes crisp-tender.

2. Put 1 sheet of phyllo dough in a cooking spray-coated 13x9-inch baking dish, then cut if needed. Use the butter-flavored spray to spritz the dough. Redo the layers 9 times. Lay the asparagus, feta cheese, and spinach on top. Cover it using a sheet of phyllo dough, then spritz it using the butter-flavored spray. Redo the process using the leftover phyllo. Slice it into 12 pieces. Let it bake for 15 minutes at 350 degrees F without cover, or until it turns golden brown.

3. To make the sauce, in a small saucepan, melt the butter. Mix in the flour until it becomes smooth, then slowly add the milk. Stir in salt, thyme, dill, and lemon juice, then boil. Let it cook and stir for 5 minutes until it becomes thick. Serve the spanakopita with the sauce.

Nutrition: Calories 112 Fat 4 Carbs 14 Protein 5

Black Bean and Corn Salsa from Red Gold

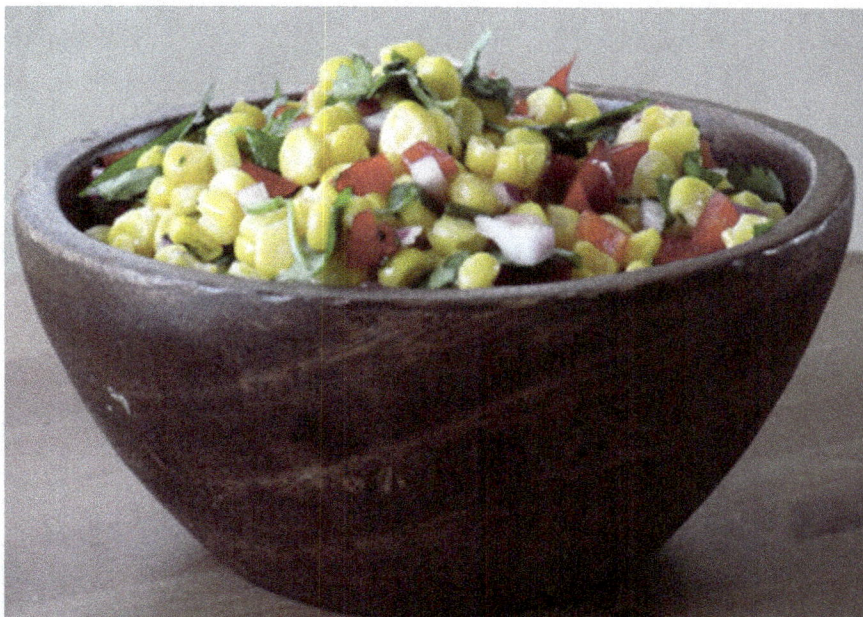

Preparation Time: 15 minutes

Cooking Time: 15 minutes

Servings: 25

Ingredients:

- 2 cans black beans, drained and rinsed

- 1 can whole kernel corn, drained

- 2 cans RED GOLD® Petite Diced Tomatoes & Green Chilies

- 1 can RED GOLD® Diced Tomatoes, drained

- 1/2 cup chopped green onions

- 2 tablespoon chopped fresh cilantro

- Salt and black pepper to taste

Directions:

1. Mix all ingredients to combine in a big bowl. Refrigerate to blend flavors for a few hours to overnight. Serve with chips or crackers.

Nutrition: Calories 65 Fat 3 Carbs 8 Protein 9

PASTA & NOODLES

Stir Fry Noodles

Preparation Time: 10 minutes

Cooking Time: 8 minutes

Servings: 4

Ingredients:

- 1 cup broccoli, chopped

- 1 cup red bell pepper, chopped

- 1 cup mushrooms, chopped

- 1 large onion, chopped

- 1 batch Stir Fry Sauce, prepared

- Salt and black pepper, to taste

- 2 cups spaghetti, cooked

- 4 garlic cloves, minced

- 2 tablespoons sesame oil

Directions:

1. Heat sesame oil in a pan over medium heat and add garlic, onions, bell pepper, broccoli, mushrooms.

2. Sauté for about 5 minutes and add spaghetti noodles and stir fry sauce.

3. Mix well and cook for 3 more minutes.

4. Dish out in plates and serve to enjoy.

Nutrition: Calories: 567 Total fat: 48g Total carbs: 6g Fiber: 4g; Net carbs: 2g Sodium: 373mg Protein: 33g

SIDE DISHES

Glazed Carrots

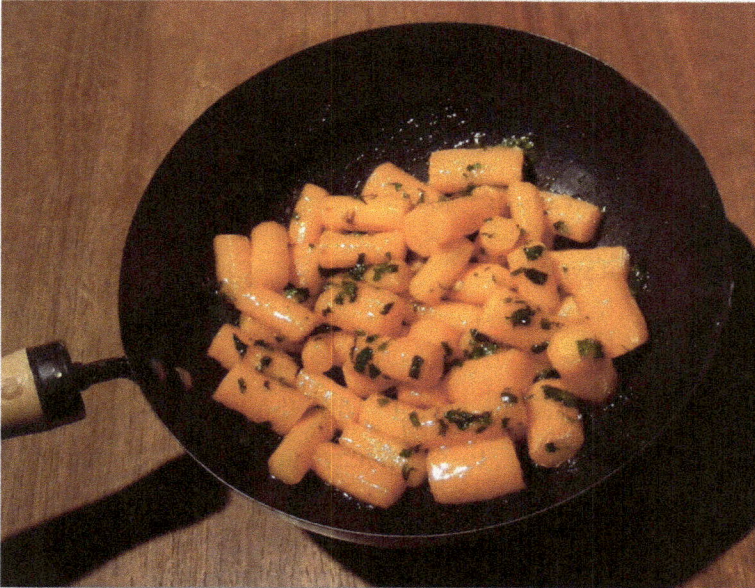

Preparation Time: 15 minutes

Cooking Time: 8 minutes

Servings: 4

Ingredients:

- 1-pound baby carrots, peeled
- 1 tablespoon Maple syrup
- 1 tablespoon olive oil
- 1 teaspoon coriander, ground
- 1/2 teaspoon minced garlic
- 1 teaspoon turmeric powder
- 1 tablespoon apple cider vinegar
- 1 tablespoon sesame seeds
- 1/2 cup of water

Directions:

1. In a bowl, mix the carrots with the maple syrup and the other Ingredients, toss and leave aside for 10 minutes.

2. Transfer the mix in the instant pot. Add water and cook on Manual mode (High pressure) for 8 minutes.

3. Then make quick pressure release.

4. Transfer the mix in the serving bowls and serve.

Nutrition: Calories: 172, Fat: 4.9, Fiber: 1.5, Carbs: 6.1, Protein: 4.

Broccoli Puree

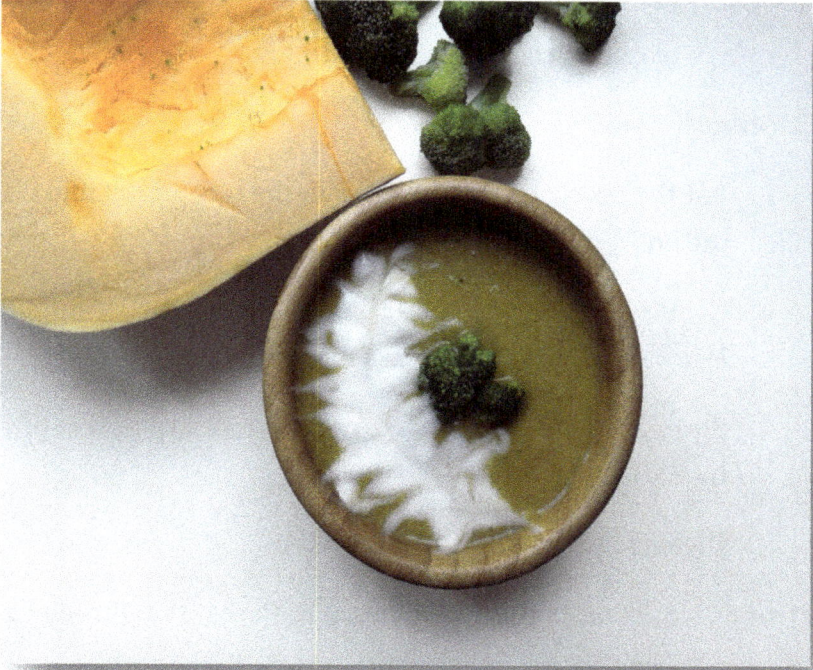

Preparation Time: 15 minutes

Cooking Time: 15 minutes

Servings: 6

Ingredients:

- 1 pound broccoli florets

- 1/3 cup almond milk

- 1 cup of water

- 1 teaspoon dried oregano

- 1/2 teaspoon coriander, ground

Directions:

1. Put the broccoli and the water in the instant pot and close the lid.

2. Cook on Manual mode (High pressure) for 15 minutes. Use natural pressure release for 10 minutes.

3. Strain, transfer to the food processor, add the rest of the Ingredients and pulse.

4. Divide between plates and serve.

Nutrition: Calories: 182, Fat: 3.8, Fiber: 4.8, Carbs: 11.1, Protein: 2

Lemon Cauliflower

Preparation Time: 7 minutes

Cooking Time: 8 minutes

Servings: 4

Ingredients:

- 1 pound cauliflower florets
- 1 teaspoon lemon zest
- 1 tablespoon lemon juice
- 1 teaspoon turmeric powder
- 1 teaspoon black pepper
- 1 teaspoon Pink salt
- 1 tablespoon fresh dill, chopped
- 1/4 cup vegetable broth
- 1 tablespoon olive oil

Directions:

1. In the instant pot, mix the cauliflower with the lemon juice, zest and the other Ingredients, close the lid and cook on Manual mode for 8 minutes.

2. Allow natural pressure release.

Nutrition: Calories: 205, Fat: 4.5, Fiber: 3.3, Carbs: 14.5, Protein: 4.2

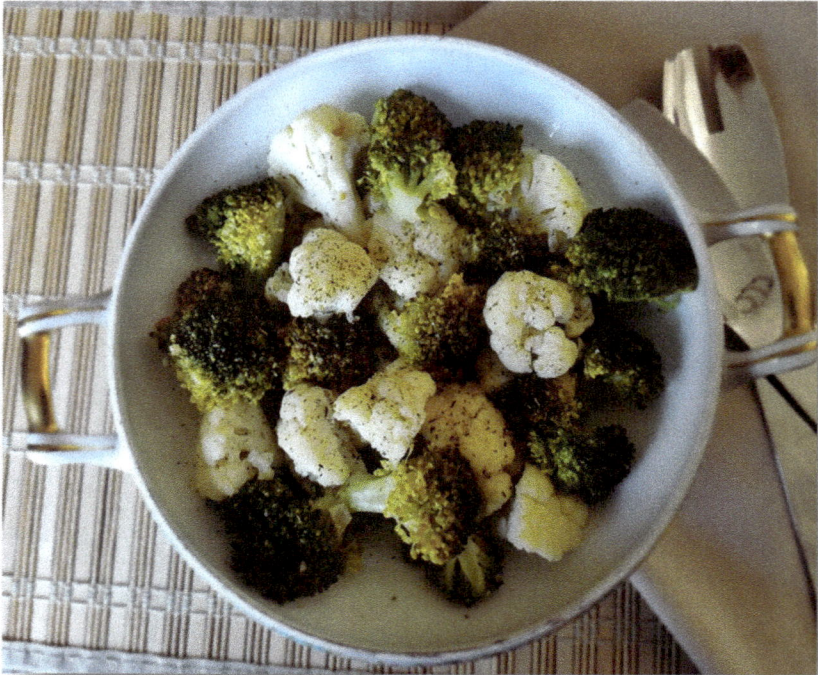

SOUP AND STEW

Vegetable Broth Sans Sodium

Preparation Time: 5 minutes

Cooking Time: 60 minutes

Servings: 1 cup

Ingredients:

- 5 sprigs of dill

- 2 freshly sliced yellow onions

- 4 chives

- 6 freshly peeled and sliced carrots

- 10 cups of water

- 4 freshly sliced celery stalks

- 3 cloves of freshly minced garlic

- 4 sprigs of parsley

Directions:

1. Put a large pot on medium heat and stir the onions. Fry the onions for 1 minute until they become fragrant. Add the garlic, celery, carrots, and dill along with the chives and parsley and cook everything. You will know that the mix is ready when it becomes fragrant.

2. Add the water and allow the mixture to boil. Reduce the heat and allow everything to cook for 45 minutes.

3. Turn off the heat. The broth will cool in about 15 minutes.

4. Strain the broth with the help of a sieve so that you have a clear vegetable broth.

5. If you are not using the broth right away, store it as ice cubes. You can store the ice cubes for a week.

Nutrition: Kcal: 362 Carbohydrates: 21 g Protein: 12 g Fat: 21 g

Amazing Chickpea and Noodle Soup

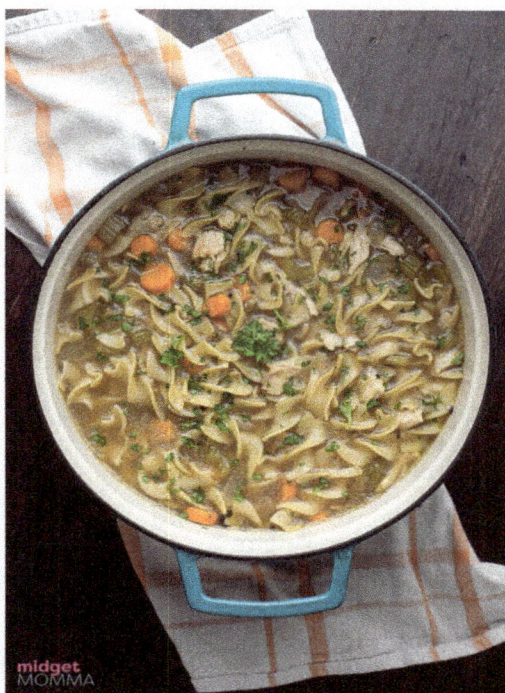

Preparation Time: 10 minutes

Cooking Time: 20 minutes

Servings: 1 cup

Ingredients:

- 1 freshly diced celery stalk
- ¼ cup of 'chicken' seasoning
- 1 cup of freshly diced onion
- 3 cloves of freshly crushed garlic
- 2 cups of cooked chickpeas
- 4 cups of vegetable broth
- Freshly chopped cilantro
- 2 freshly cubed medium-size potatoes
- Salt
- 2 freshly sliced carrots
- ½ teaspoon of dried thyme
- Pepper
- 2 cups of water
- 6 ounces of gluten-free spaghetti
- 'Chicken' seasoning
- 1 tablespoon of garlic powder
- 2 teaspoons of sea salt
- 1 1/3 cup of nutritional yeast

- 3 tablespoons of onion powder

- 1 teaspoon of oregano

- ½ teaspoon of turmeric

- 1 ½ tablespoons of dried basil

Directions:

1. Put a pot on medium heat and sauté the onion. It will soften within 3 minutes.

2. Add celery, potato, and carrots and sauté for another 3 minutes

3. Add the 'chicken' seasoning to the garlic, thyme, water, and vegetable broth.

4. Simmer the mix on medium-high heat. Cook the veggies for about 20 minutes until they soften.

5. Add the cooked pasta and chickpeas.

6. Add salt and pepper to taste.

7. Put the fresh cilantro on top and enjoy the fresh soup!

Nutrition: Kcal: 405 Carbohydrates: 1 g Protein: 19 g Fat: 38 g

Sweet Potato, Corn and Jalapeno Bisque

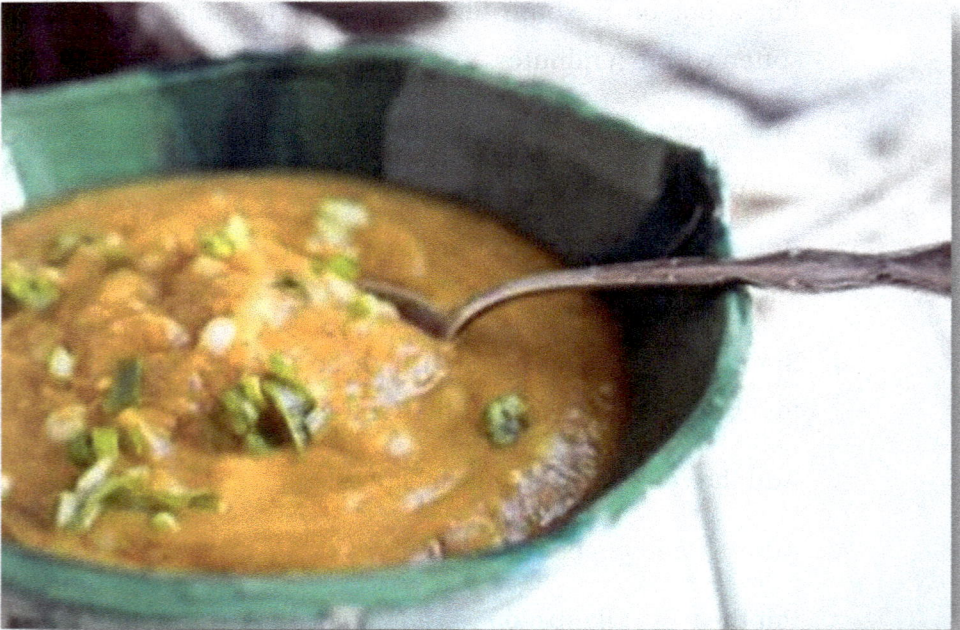

Preparation Time: 10 minutes

Cooking Time: 15 minutes

Servings: 4

Ingredients:

- 4 ears corn
- 1 seeded and chopped jalapeno
- 4 cups vegetable broth
- 1 tablespoon olive oil
- 3 peeled and cubed sweet potatoes
- 1 chopped onion
- ½ tablespoon salt
- ¼ teaspoon black pepper
- 1 minced garlic clove

Directions:

1. In a pan, heat the oil over medium flame and sauté onion and garlic in it and cook for around 3 minutes. Put broth and sweet potatoes in it and bring it to boil. Reduce the flame and cook it for an additional 10 minutes.

2. Remove it from the stove and blend it with a blender. Again, put it on the stove and add corn, jalapeno, salt, and black pepper and serve it.

Nutrition: Carbohydrates 31g Protein 6g Fats 4g Sugar 11g.

Creamy Pea Soup with Olive Pesto

Preparation Time: 20 minutes

Cooking Time: 20 minutes

Servings: 4

Ingredients:

- 1 grated carrot

- 1 rinsed chopped leek

- 1 minced garlic clove

- 2 tablespoons olive oil

- 1 stem fresh thyme leaves

- 15 ounces rinsed and drained peas

- ½ tablespoon salt

- ¼ teaspoon ground black pepper

- 2 ½ cups vegetable broth

- ¼ cup parsley leaves

- 1 ¼ cups pitted green olives

- 1 teaspoon drained capers

- 1 garlic clove

Directions:

1. Take a pan with oil and put it over medium flame and whisk garlic, leek, thyme, and carrot in it. Cook it for around 4 minutes.

2. Add broth, peas, salt, and pepper and increase the heat. When it starts boiling, lower down the heat and cook it with a lid on for around 15 minutes and remove from heat and blend it.

3. For making pesto whisk parsley, olives, capers, and garlic and blend it in a way that it has little chunks. Top the soup with the scoop of olive pesto.

Nutrition: Carbohydrates 23g Protein 6g Fats 15g Sugar 4g Calories 230.

Spinach Soup with Dill and Basil

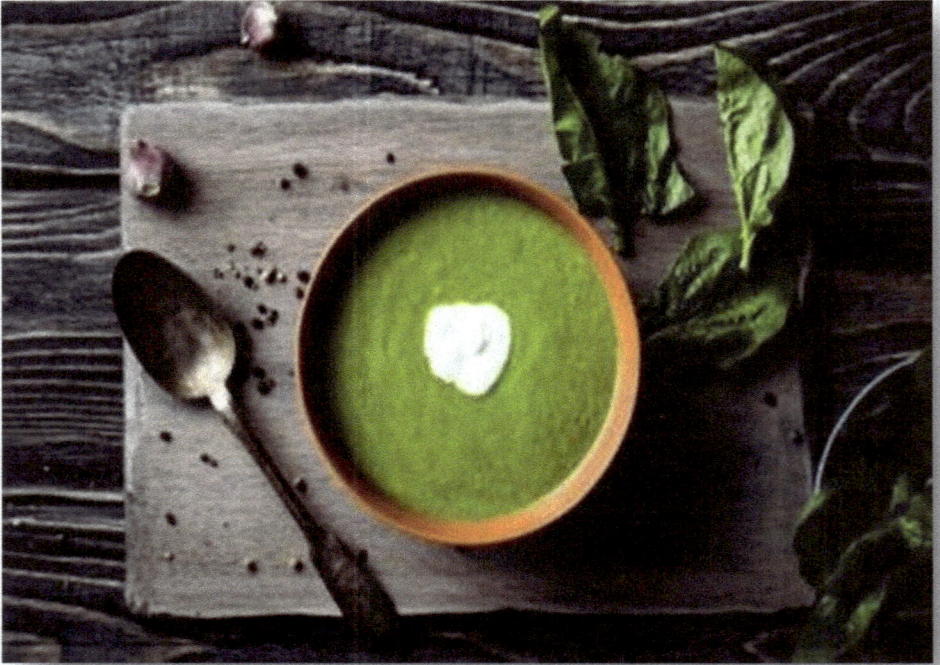

Preparation Time: 10 minutes

Cooking Time: 25 minutes

Servings: 8

Ingredients:

- 1 pound peeled and diced potatoes

- 1 tablespoon minced garlic

- 1 teaspoon dry mustard

- 6 cups vegetable broth

- 20 ounces chopped frozen spinach

- 2 cups chopped onion

- 1 ½ tablespoons salt

- ½ cup minced dill

- 1 cup basil

- ½ teaspoon ground black pepper

Directions:

1. Whisk onion, garlic, potatoes, broth, mustard, and salt in a pan and cook it over medium flame. When it starts boiling, low down the heat and cover it with the lid and cook for 20 minutes.

2. Add the remaining ingredients in it and blend it and cook it for few more minutes and serve it.

Nutrition: Carbohydrates 12g Protein 13g Fats 1g Calories 165

Roasted Red Pepper and Butternut Squash Soup

Preparation Time: 10 minutes

Cooking Time: 45 minutes

Servings: 6

Ingredients:

- 1 small butternut squash
- 1 tablespoon olive oil
- 1 teaspoon sea salt
- 2 red bell peppers
- 1 yellow onion
- 1 head garlic
- 2 cups water, or vegetable broth
- Zest and juice of 1 lime
- 1 to 2 tablespoons tahini
- Pinch cayenne pepper
- ½ teaspoon ground coriander

- ½ teaspoon ground cumin

- Toasted squash seeds (optional)

Directions:

1. Preparing the ingredients.

2. Preheat the oven to 350°f.

3. Prepare the squash for roasting by cutting it in half lengthwise, scooping out the seeds, and poking some holes in the flesh with a fork. Reserve the seeds if desired.

4. Rub a small amount of oil over the flesh and skin, then rub with a bit of sea salt and put the halves skin-side down in a large baking dish. Put it in the oven while you prepare the rest of the vegetables.

5. Prepare the peppers the exact same way, except they do not need to be poked.

6. Slice the onion in half and rub oil on the exposed faces. Slice the top off the head of garlic and rub oil on the exposed flesh.

7. After the squash has cooked for 20 minutes, add the peppers, onion, and garlic, and roast for another 20 minutes. Optionally, you can toast the squash seeds by putting them in the oven in a separate baking dish 10 to 15 minutes before the vegetables are finished.

8. Keep a close eye on them. When the vegetables are cooked, take them out and let them cool before handling them. The squash will be very soft when poked with a fork.

9. Scoop the flesh out of the squash skin into a large pot (if you have an immersion blender) or into a blender.

10. Chop the pepper roughly, remove the onion skin and chop the onion roughly, and squeeze the garlic cloves out of the head, all into the pot or blender. Add the water, the lime zest and juice, and the tahini. Purée the soup, adding more water if you like, to your desired consistency. Season with the salt, cayenne, coriander, and cumin. Serve garnished with toasted squash seeds (if using).

Nutrition: Calories: 156 Protein: 4g Total fat: 7g Saturated fat: 11g Carbohydrates: 22g Fiber: 5g

SMOOTHIES AND BEVERAGES

Kale Smoothie

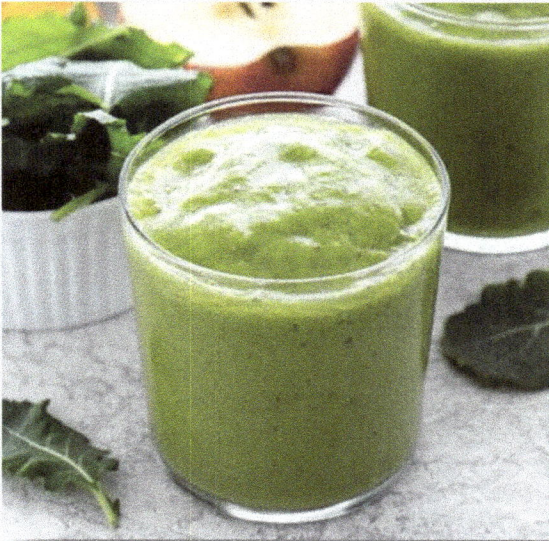

Preparation Time: 5 minutes

Cooking Time: 0 minutes

Servings: 2

Ingredients:

- 2 cups chopped kale leaves

- 1 banana, peeled

- 1 cup frozen strawberries

- 1 cup unsweetened almond milk

- 4 Medjool dates, pitted and chopped

Directions:

1. Put all the ingredients in a food processor, then blitz until glossy and smooth.

2. Serve immediately or chill in the refrigerator for an hour before serving.

Nutrition: Calories: 663 Fat: 10.0g Carbs: 142.5g Fiber: 19.0g Protein: 17.4g

Hot Tropical Smoothie

Preparation Time: 5 minutes

Cooking Time: 0 minutes

Servings: 4

Ingredients:

- 1 cup frozen mango chunks

- 1 cup frozen pineapple chunks

- 1 small tangerine, peeled and pitted

- 2 cups spinach leaves

- 1 cup coconut water

- ¼ teaspoon cayenne pepper, optional

Directions:

1. Add all the ingredients in a food processor, then blitz until the mixture is smooth and combine well.

2. Serve immediately or chill in the refrigerator for an hour before serving.

Nutrition: Calories: 283 Fat: 1.9g Carbs: 67.9g Fiber: 10.4g Protein: 6.4g

BREAD RECIPES

Delicious Cheese Bread

Preparation Time: 10 Minutes

Cooking Time: 35 Minutes

Servings: 12

Ingredients:

- Eggs – 2

- All-purpose flour – 2 cups

- Butter – 1/2 cup, melted

- Buttermilk – 1 cup

- Baking soda – 1/2 teaspoon.

- Baking powder – 1/2 teaspoon.

- Sugar – 1 teaspoon.

- Cheddar cheese – 1 cup, shredded

- Salt– 1/2 teaspoon.

Directions:

1. Preheat the oven for 350 F. In a large mixing bowl, mix flour, baking soda, baking powder, sugar, cheese, pepper, and salt.

2. In a small bowl, beat eggs with buttermilk, and butter. Add egg mixture to the flour mixture and mix well.

3. Transfer mixture into the greased 9*5-inch loaf pan and bake in preheated oven for 35-40 minutes.

4. Allow to cool for 15 minutes. Slice and serve.

Nutrition: Calories 202, Carbs 17.6g, Fat 11.9g, Protein 6.2g

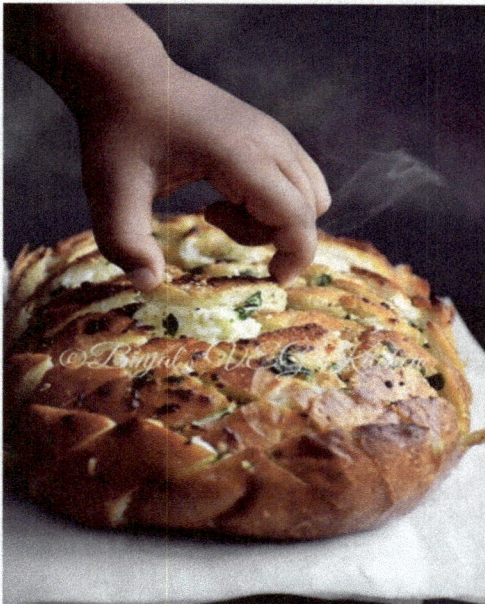

Strawberry Bread

Preparation Time: 15 Minutes

Cooking Time: 60 Minutes

Servings: 10

Ingredients:

- Eggs – 2

- All-purpose flour – 2 cups

- Vanilla – 1 teaspoon.

- Vegetable oil – 1/2 cup

- Baking soda – 1 teaspoon.

- Cinnamon – 1/2 teaspoon.

- Brown sugar – 1/2 cup

- White sugar – 1/2 cup

- Fresh strawberries – 2 1/4 cups, chopped

- Salt – 1/2 teaspoon.

Directions:

1. Preheat the oven to 350 F. Grease 9.5-inch loaf pan and set aside.

2. In a mixing bowl, mix together flour, baking soda, cinnamon, brown sugar, white sugar, and salt.

3. In a separate bowl, beat eggs, vanilla, and oil. Stir in strawberries.

4. Add flour mixture to the egg mixture and stir until well combined.

5. Pour batter into the prepared loaf pan and bake in preheated oven for 50-60 minutes.

6. Allow to cool for 10-15 minutes. Slice and serve.

Nutrition: Calories 364, Carbs 40.1g, Fat 21.g, Protein 4.2g

Almond Bread

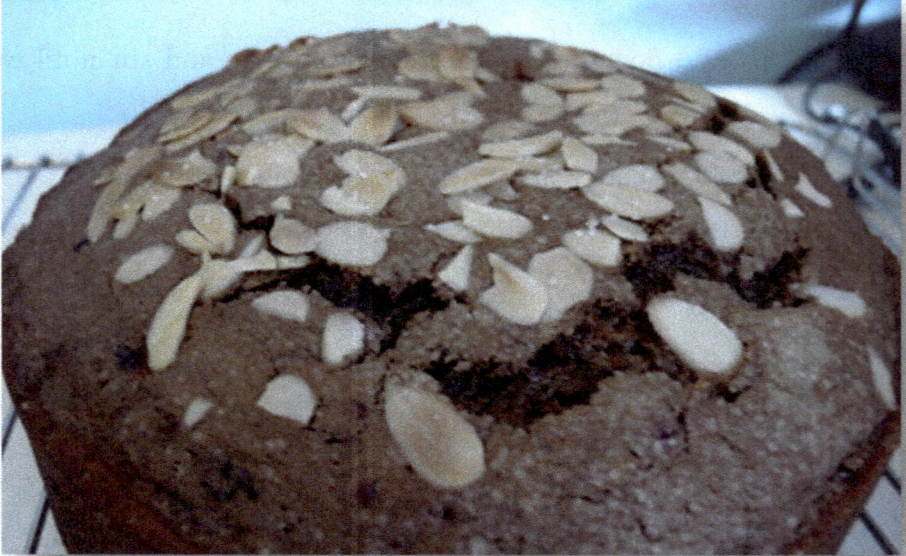

Preparation Time: 10 Minutes

Cooking Time: 30 Minutes

Servings: 20

Ingredients:

- Eggs – 6, separated

- Cream of tartar – 1/4 teaspoon.

- Baking powder – 3 teaspoon.

- Butter – 4 tablespoons, melted

- Almond flour – 1 1/2 cups

- Salt – 1/4 teaspoon.

Directions:

1. Preheat the oven to 375 F. Grease 8*4-inch loaf pan with butter and set aside. Add egg whites and cream of tartar in a large bowl and beat until soft peaks form.

2. Add almond flour, baking powder, egg yolks, butter, and salt in a food processor and process until combined.

3. Add 1/3 of egg white mixture into the almond flour mixture and process until combined. Now add remaining egg white mixture and process gently to combine.

4. Pour batter into the prepared loaf pan and bake for 30 minutes. Slice and serve.

Nutrition: Calories 52, Carbs 1g, Fat 4g, Protein 2g

SAUCES, DRESSINGS, AND DIPS

Satay Sauce

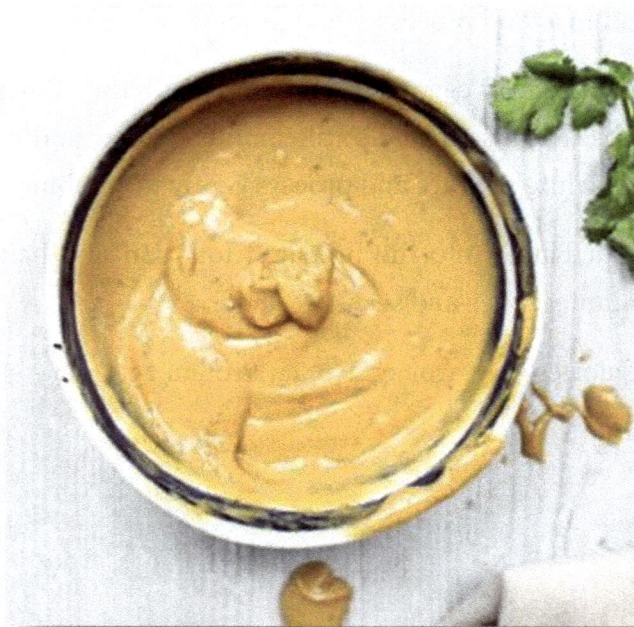

Preparation Time: 5 minutes

Cooking Time: 8 minutes

Servings: 2

Ingredients:

- ½ yellow onion, diced

- 3 garlic cloves, minced

- 1 fresh red chile, thinly sliced (optional)

- 1-inch (2.5-cm) piece fresh ginger, peeled and minced

- ¼ cup smooth peanut butter

- 2 tablespoons coconut aminos

- 1 (13.5-ounce / 383-g) can unsweetened coconut milk

- ¼ teaspoon freshly ground black pepper

- ¼ teaspoon salt (optional)

Directions:

1. Heat a large nonstick skillet over medium-high heat until hot.

2. Add the onion, garlic cloves, chile (if desired), and ginger to the skillet, and sauté for 2 minutes.

3. Pour in the peanut butter and coconut aminos and stir well. Add the coconut milk, black pepper, and salt (if

desired) and continue whisking, or until the sauce is just beginning to bubble and thicken.

4. Remove the sauce from the heat to a bowl. Taste and adjust the seasoning if necessary.

Nutrition: Calories: 322 Fat: 28.8g Carbs: 9.4gProtein: 6.3gFiber: 1.8g

SALADS RECIPES

Cashew Siam Salad

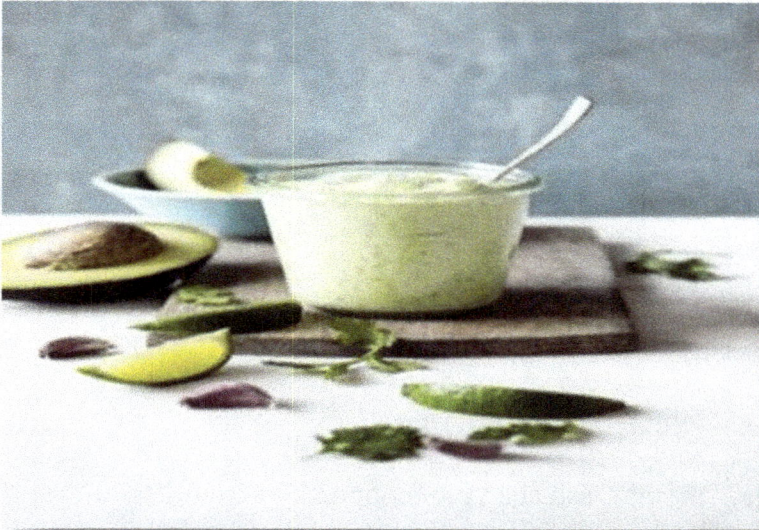

Preparation Time: 10 minutes

Cooking Time: 3 minutes

Servings: 4

Ingredients:

Salad:

- 4 cups baby spinach, rinsed, drained
- ½ cup pickled red cabbage

Dressing:

- 1-inch piece ginger, finely chopped
- 1 tsp. chili garlic paste
- 1 tbsp. soy sauce
- ½ tbsp. rice vinegar
- 1 tbsp. sesame oil
- 3 tbsp. avocado oil

Toppings:

- ½ cup raw cashews, unsalted
- ¼ cup fresh cilantro, chopped

Directions:

1. Put the spinach and red cabbage in a large bowl. Toss to combine and set the salad aside.

2. Toast the cashews in a frying pan over medium-high heat, stirring occasionally until the cashews are golden brown. This should take about 3 minutes. Turn off the heat and set the frying pan aside.

3. Mix all the dressing ingredients in medium-sized bowl and use a spoon to mix them into a smooth dressing.

4. Pour the dressing over the spinach salad and top with the toasted cashews.

5. Toss the salad to combine all ingredients and transfer the large bowl to the fridge. Allow the salad to chill for up to one hour – doing so will guarantee a better flavor. Alternatively, the salad can be served right away, topped with the optional cilantro. Enjoy!

Nutrition: Calories 160 Total Fat 12.9g Saturated Fat 2.4g Cholesterol 0mg Sodium 265mg Total Carbohydrate 9.1g Dietary Fiber 2.1g Total Sugars 1.4g Protein 4.1g Vitamin D 0mcg Calcium 45mg Iron 2mg Potassium 344mg

FRUIT SALAD RECIPES

Ambrosia with Pineapple

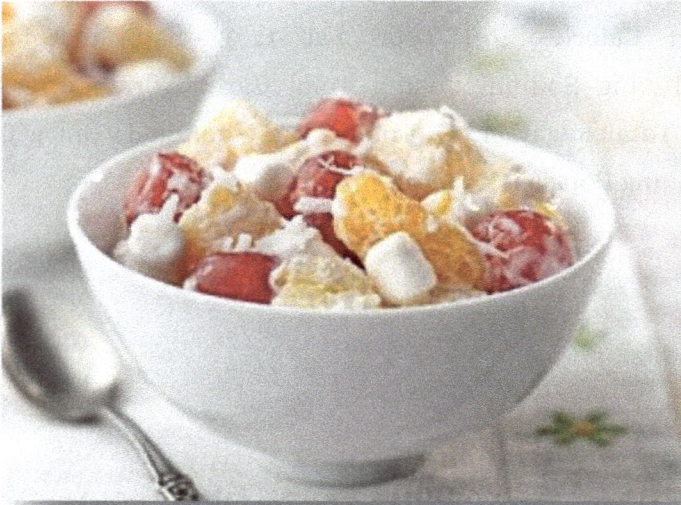

Preparation Time: 30 Minutes

Cooking Time: 15 Minutes

Servings: 4

Ingredients:

- Orange zest, two teaspoons

- Tofu, soft, pureed, one half cup

- Orange juice, three tablespoons

- Lemon juice, one third cup

- Cornstarch, one tablespoon

- Coconut, unsweetened shredded, one half cup

- Grapes, one cup

- Sugar, three tablespoons

- Strawberries, sliced, one cup

- Orange slices, one cup

- Apples, fresh sliced, one cup

- Pineapple, fresh chopped, one cup

Directions:

1. Use a large-sized bowl to assemble the fruits together and put it in the refrigerator.

2. In a small saucepan, mix together the lemon juice with the cornstarch and keep stirring until they are well mixed.

3. Add in the orange juice and the sugar and place the saucepan over medium-high heat. Cook the mix for five to

ten minutes while the mixture gets thicker. Keep stirring constantly.

4. When the mixture is thick, then take the saucepan off of the heat and let it get completely cool.

5. When the mixture in the saucepan has cooled completely, then blends in the orange zest and the pureed tofu.

6. Allow this bowl of mix to rest in the refrigerator for one hour until it becomes chilled. Pour the dressing over the fruit before serving.

Nutrition: Calories: 257 Protein: 8g Fat: 8g Carbs: 44

ENTRÉES

BLT Panini with Eggplant "Bacon"

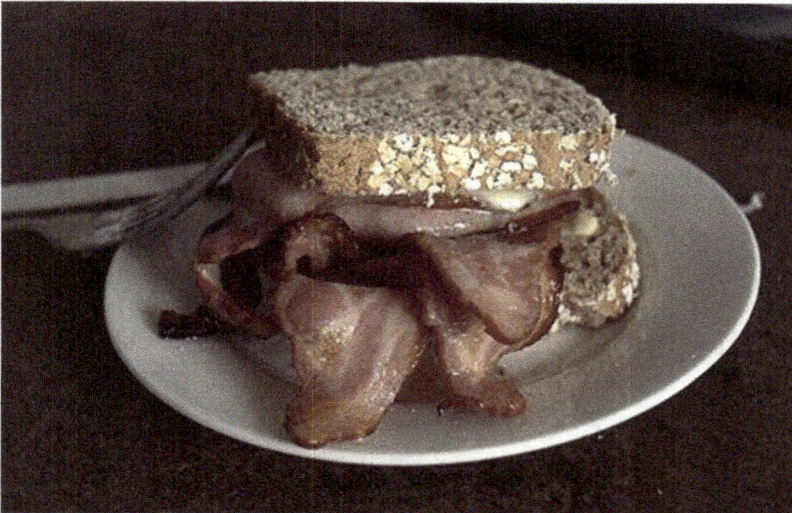

Preparation Time: 10 minutes

Cooking Time: 25 minutes

Servings: 2

Ingredients:

- Eggplant, medium – 1
- Tomato, sliced into rounds – 1
- Cucumber, medium, sliced into rounds - .5
- Arugula lettuce - .5 cup
- Vegan mayonnaise – 2 tablespoons
- Ciabatta buns – 2
- Tamari sauce – 1 tablespoon
- Sea salt - 1.25 teaspoon
- Maple syrup – 1 teaspoon
- Olive oil – 1 tablespoon
- Paprika, smoked – 1 teaspoon
- Black pepper, ground - .25 teaspoon

Directions:

1. Peel the eggplant, slice it into rounds, and soak it in salt water made with one teaspoon of the sea salt. Allow the eggplant to sit in the saltwater for ten minutes. Remove the eggplant from the saltwater once soaked for the ten-minute duration and then pat it dry with a clean kitchen towel.

2. In a small bowl whisk together the tamari sauce, sea salt, maple syrup, olive oil, smoked paprika, and ground black pepper.

3. Place the eggplant slices on a baking sheet. Use the combined sauce and with a pastry brush cover it over the eggplant slices on all sides. Bake the eggplant slices until tender, for about twenty minutes in a large oven preheated to a temperature of three-hundred- and seventy-five-degrees Fahrenheit.

4. Once the eggplant is done cooking prepare your panini. Begin by slicing the ciabatta rolls in half. Spread the inside of the rolls with vegan mayonnaise before topping with the eggplant "bacon," tomato, cucumber, and lastly the arugula. Close the sandwich with the top half of the rolls.

5. Wrap the sandwiches in aluminum foil before placing them in a panini grill. However, if you do not have a panini grill, you can do this in a large skillet by weighing down the sandwich with a heavy pan, such as a small cast iron pan.

6. Allow the sandwiches to grill until warm and crispy, about three to four minutes. Enjoy the sandwich immediately, or leave it in the aluminum foil to take on-the-go.

Nutrition: Number of Calories in Individual **Servings:** 364 Protein Grams: 10 Fat Grams: 14 Total Carbohydrates Grams: 51 Net Carbohydrates Grams: 41

GRAINS AND BEANS

Veggie Barley Bowl

Preparation Time: 10 minutes

Cooking Time: 1 hour 11 minutes

Servings: 8

Ingredients:

- 1 cup barley

- 3 cups low-sodium vegetable broth

- 2 cups sliced mushrooms

- 2 cups broccoli florets

- 1 cup snow peas, trimmed

- ½ cup sliced scallion

- ¼ cup chopped green bell pepper

- ¼ cup chopped red bell pepper

- 1 cup bean sprouts

- ¼ cup soy sauce

- ¼ cup water

- ¼ teaspoon ground ginger

- 1 tablespoon cornstarch, mixed with 2 tablespoons cold water

Directions:

1. In a saucepan over medium heat, place the barley and vegetable stock. Cover and cook for 1 hour.

2. Combine all the vegetables, except for the bean sprouts, in a large pot with the soy sauce, water and ginger. Cook for 5 minutes, stirring constantly.

3. Add the bean sprouts and cook, stirring, for another 5 minutes. Add the cornstarch mixture and cook for about 1 minute, stirring, or until thickened.

4. Remove from the heat. Toss the vegetables with the cooked barley.

5. Serve hot.

Nutrition: Calories: 190 Fat: 2.6g Carbs: 35.7g Protein: 5.9g Fiber: 6.9g

DRINKS

Chocolate Banana Shake

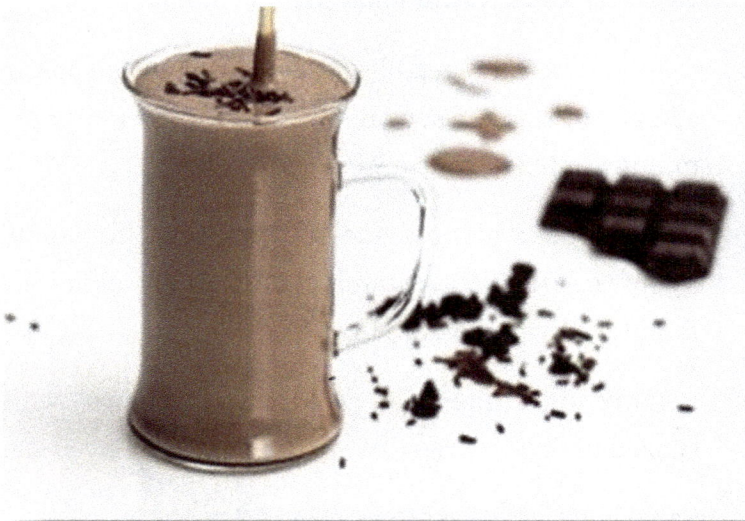

Preparation Time: 10 minutes

Cooking Time: 10 minutes

Servings: 2

Ingredients:

- 2 medium frozen bananas, peeled
- 4 dates, pitted
- 4 tablespoons peanut butter
- 4 tablespoons rolled oats
- 2 tablespoons cacao powder
- 2 tablespoons chia seeds
- 2 cups unsweetened soymilk

Directions:

1. Place all the ingredients in a high-speed blender and pulse until creamy.

2. Pour into two glasses and serve immediately.

Nutrition: Calories: 502 Fat: 4g Protein: 11g Sugar: 9g

Fruity Tofu Smoothie

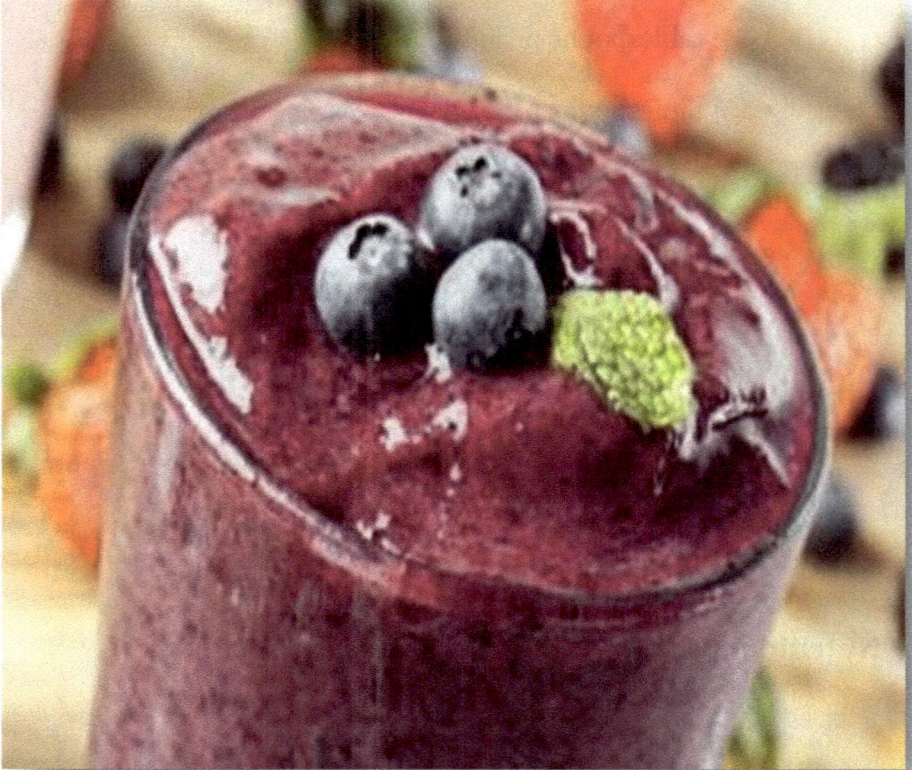

Preparation Time: 10 minutes

Cooking Time: 10 minutes

Servings: 2

Ingredients:

- 12 ounces silken tofu, pressed and drained
- 2 medium bananas, peeled
- 1½ cups fresh blueberries
- 1 tablespoon maple syrup
- 1½ cups unsweetened soymilk
- ¼ cup ice cubes

Directions:

1. Place all the ingredients in a high-speed blender and pulse until creamy.
2. Pour into two glasses and serve immediately.

Nutrition: Calories 235 Carbohydrates: 1.9g Protein: 14.3g Fat: 18.9g

Protein Latte

Preparation Time: 10 minutes

Cooking Time: 10 minutes

Servings: 2

Ingredients:

- 2 cups hot brewed coffee

- 1¼ cups coconut milk

- 2 teaspoons coconut oil

- 2 scoops unsweetened vegan vanilla protein powder

Directions:

1. Place all the ingredients in a high-speed blender and pulse until creamy.

2. Pour into two serving mugs and serve immediately.

Nutrition: Calories 483 Carbs: 5.2g Protein: 45.2g Fat: 31.2g

Thai Iced Tea

Preparation Time: 5 minutes

Cooking Time: 10 minutes

Servings: 4

Ingredients:

- 4 cups of water

- 1 can of light coconut milk (14 oz.)

- ¼ cup of maple syrup

- ¼ cup of muscovado sugar

- 1 teaspoon of vanilla extract

- 2 tablespoons of loose-leaf black tea

Directions:

1. In a large saucepan, over medium heat bring the water to a boil.

2. Turn off the heat and add in the tea, cover and let steep for five minutes.

3. Strain the tea into a bowl or jug. Add the maple syrup, muscovado sugar, and vanilla extract. Give it a good whisk to blend all the ingredients together.

4. Set in the refrigerator to chill. Upon serving, pour ¾ of the tea into each glass, top with coconut milk and stir.

Tips:

Add a shot of dark rum to turn this iced tea into a cocktail.

You could substitute the coconut milk for almond or rice milk too.

Nutrition: Calories 844 Carbohydrates: 2.3g Protein: 21.6g Fat: 83.1g

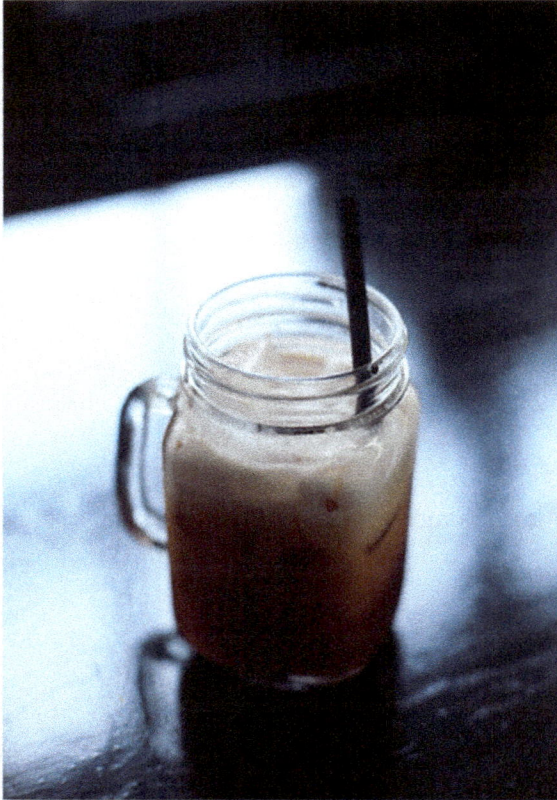

DESSERTS

Chocolate and Avocado Pudding

Preparation Time: 3 hours and 10 minutes

Cooking Time: 0 minute

Servings: 1

Ingredients:

- 1 small avocado, pitted, peeled

- 1 small banana, mashed

- 1/3 cup cocoa powder, unsweetened

- 1 tablespoon cacao nibs, unsweetened

- 1/4 cup maple syrup

- 1/3 cup coconut cream

Directions:

1. Add avocado in a food processor along with cream and then pulse for 2 minutes until smooth.

2. Add remaining ingredients, blend until mixed, and then tip the pudding in a container.

3. Cover the container with a plastic wrap; it should touch the pudding and refrigerate for 3 hours.

4. Serve straight away.

Nutrition: Calories: 87 Cal Fat: 7 g Carbs: 9 g Protein: 1.5 g Fiber: 3.2 g

Chocolate Avocado Ice Cream

Preparation Time: 1 hour and 10 minutes

Cooking Time: 0 minute

Servings: 2

Ingredients:

- 4.5 ounces avocado, peeled, pitted

- 1/2 cup cocoa powder, unsweetened

- 1 tablespoon vanilla extract, unsweetened

- 1/2 cup and 2 tablespoons maple syrup

- 13.5 ounces coconut milk, unsweetened

- 1/2 cup water

Directions:

1. Add avocado in a food processor along with milk and then pulse for 2 minutes until smooth.

2. Add remaining ingredients, blend until mixed, and then tip the pudding in a freezer-proof container.

3. Place the container in a freezer and chill for freeze for 4 hours until firm, whisking every 20 minutes after 1 hour.

4. Serve straight away.

Nutrition: Calories: 80.7 Cal Fat: 7.1 g Carbs: 6 g Protein: 0.6 g Fiber: 2 g

Watermelon Mint Popsicles

Preparation Time: 8 hours and 5 minutes

Cooking Time: 0 minute

Servings: 8

Ingredients:

- 20 mint leaves, diced

- 6 cups watermelon chunks

- 3 tablespoons lime juice

Directions:

1. Add watermelon in a food processor along with lime juice and then pulse for 15 seconds until smooth.

2. Pass the watermelon mixture through a strainer placed over a bowl, remove the seeds and then stir mint into the collected watermelon mixture.

3. Take eight Popsicle molds, pour in prepared watermelon mixture, and freeze for 2 hours until slightly firm.

4. Then insert popsicle sticks and continue freezing for 6 hours until solid.

5. Serve straight away

Nutrition: Calories: 90 Cal Fat: 0 g Carbs: 23 g Protein: 0 g Fiber: 0 g

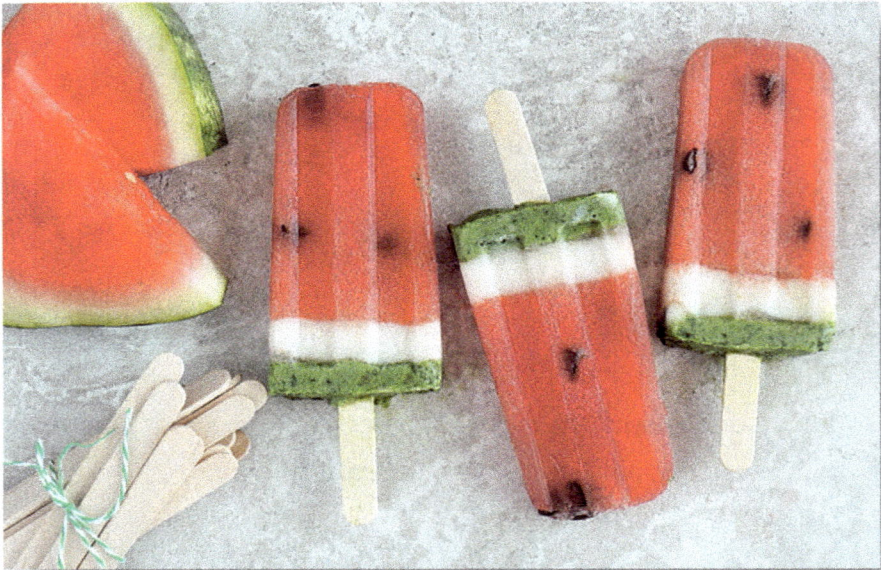

Brownie Energy Bites

Preparation Time: 1 hour and 10 minutes

Cooking Time: 0 minute

Servings: 2

Ingredients:

- 1/2 cup walnuts

- 1 cup Medjool dates, chopped

- 1/2 cup almonds

- 1/8 teaspoon salt

- 1/2 cup shredded coconut flakes

- 1/3 cup and 2 teaspoons cocoa powder, unsweetened

Directions:

1. Place almonds and walnuts in a food processor and pulse for 3 minutes until the dough starts to come together.

2. Add remaining ingredients, reserving ¼ cup of coconut and pulse for 2 minutes until incorporated.

3. Shape the mixture into balls, roll them in remaining coconut until coated, and refrigerate for 1 hour.

4. Serve straight away

Nutrition: Calories: 174.6 Cal Fat: 8.1 g Carbs: 25.5 g Protein: 4.1 g
Fiber: 4.4 g

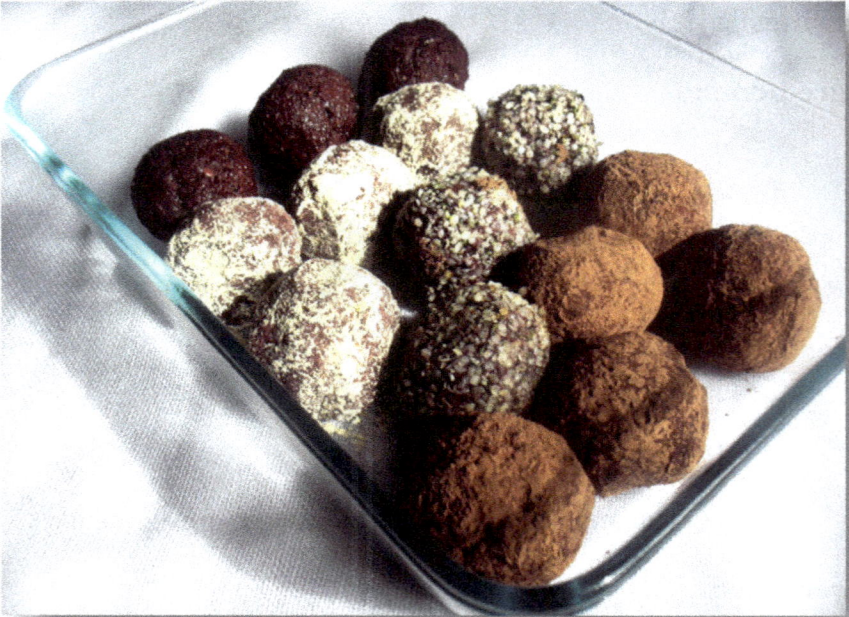

Salted Caramel Chocolate Cups

Preparation Time: 5 minutes

Cooking Time: 2 minutes

Servings: 12

Ingredients:

- ¼ teaspoon sea salt granules

- 1 cup dark chocolate chips, unsweetened

- 2 teaspoons coconut oil

- 6 tablespoons caramel sauce

Directions:

1. Take a heatproof bowl, add chocolate chips and oil, stir until mixed, then microwave for 1 minute until melted, stir chocolate and continue heating in the microwave for 30 seconds.

2. Take twelve mini muffin tins, line them with muffin liners, spoon a little bit of chocolate mixture into the tins, spread the chocolate in the bottom and along the sides, and freeze for 10 minutes until set.

3. Then fill each cup with ½ tablespoon of caramel sauce, cover with remaining chocolate and freeze for another 2salto minutes until set.

4. When ready to eat, peel off liner from the cup, sprinkle with sauce, and serve.

Nutrition: Calories: 80 Cal Fat: 5 g Carbs: 10 g Protein: 1 g Fiber: 0.5 g

Vanilla Cheesecake

Preparation Time: 3 hours 20 minutes

Cooking Time: 0 minute

Servings: 10

Ingredients:

- 1 tbsp. vanilla extract,

- 2 ½ tbsp. lemon juice

- ½ c. coconut oil

- 1/8 t. stevia powder

- 6 tbsp. coconut milk

- 1 ½ c. blanched almonds soaked

Crust:

- 2 tbsp. coconut oil

- 1 ½ c. almonds

Directions:

For the Crust:

1. In a food processor, add the almonds and coconut oil and pulse until crumbles start to form.

2. Line a 7-inch spring form pan with parchment paper and firmly press the crust into the bottom.

3. For the Sauce:

4. Bring a saucepan of water to a boil and soak the almonds for 2 hours. Drain and shake to dry.

5. Next, add the almonds to the food processor and blend until completely smooth.

6. Add vanilla, lemon, coconut oil, stevia, and coconut milk and blend until smooth.

7. Pour over the crust and freeze overnight or for a minimum of 3 hours.

8. Serve and enjoy.

Nutrition: Calories: 267 Fat: 13g Fiber: 14g Carbs: 17g Protein: 10g

OTHER RECIPES

Tahini Miso Dressing

Preparation Time: 10 minutes

Cooking Time: 0 minute

Servings: 2

Ingredients:

- ¼ cup tahini

- 1 tablespoon tamari or low-sodium soy sauce

- 1 tablespoon white miso

- 1 tablespoon freshly squeezed lemon juice

- 1 tablespoon maple syrup or honey

- ¼ cup warm water

- Freshly ground black pepper

Directions:

1. In a small bowl, whisk the tahini, tamari, miso, lemon juice, and maple syrup together. Whisk in the water and

black pepper. Store in an airtight container in the refrigerator for up to six months.

Nutrition: Calories: 76 Fat: 6g Carbs: 5g Protein: 2g

Balsamic Roasted Tomatoes

Preparation Time: 10 minutes

Cooking Time: 4 hours

Servings: 6

Ingredients:

- 6 medium tomatoes or 1 pint cherry tomatoes

- ¼ cup, plus 1 tablespoon olive oil

- Kosher salt

- Freshly ground black pepper

- 2 teaspoons balsamic vinegar

Directions:

1. Preheat the oven to 300°F. Put your rimmed baking sheet with parchment paper.

2. Wash and dry the tomatoes and halve them crosswise. Put them cut-side up on the parchment paper, and drizzle them with ¼ cup of olive oil, allowing the oil to pool on the parchment paper. Sprinkle with the salt and pepper.

3. Roast for 3 to 4 hours, or until the edges of the tomatoes are puckered and the cut surface is a little dry.

4. Sprinkle with the balsamic vinegar and let cool on the baking sheet.

5. Pack into an airtight container and pour any excess oil from the parchment paper on top. Add the remaining 1 tablespoon of oil to the container. Seal and refrigerate for up to one month.

Nutrition: Calories: 123 Fat: 12g Carbs: 5g Protein: 1g

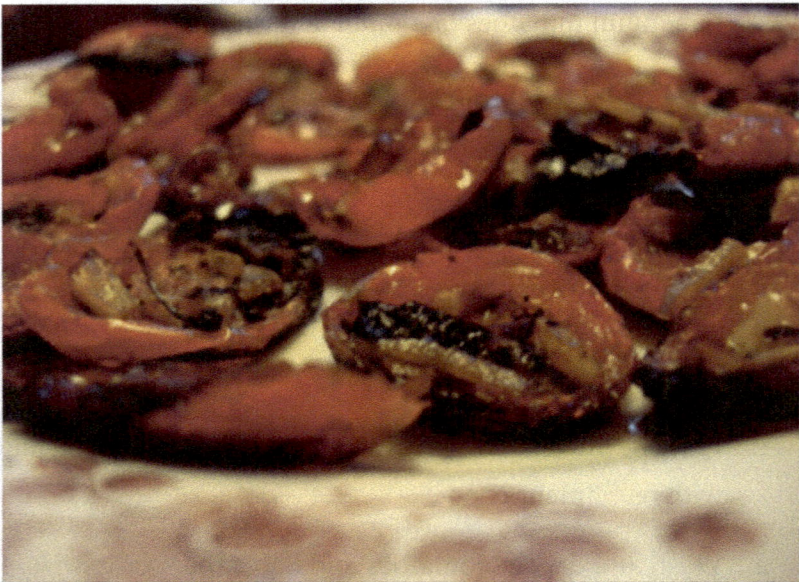

White Sauce (Béchamel)

Preparation Time: 10 minutes

Cooking Time: 12 minutes

Servings: 2

Ingredients:

- 6 tablespoons olive oil

- 4 cups soymilk or any other non-dairy milk of your choice

- 5 tablespoons all-purpose flour

- Sea salt to taste

- Black pepper to taste

Directions:

1. Place a heavy pot over a medium heat. Add oil. When the oil is heated, add sifted flour into the pan. Stir constantly for about a minute. It will begin to change colour; be careful not to burn it!

2. Pour in the milk, stirring constantly. Keep stirring until thick.

3. Simmer until the thickness you desire is nearly achieved. This is because the sauce thickens further as it cools.

4. Turn off the heat. Add salt, pepper and any other herbs and spices if you desire.

Nutrition: Calories: 68 Fat: 2 g Carbs: 1.5 g Protein: 5 g

www.ingramcontent.com/pod-product-compliance
Lightning Source LLC
Chambersburg PA
CBHW062118040426
42336CB00041B/1821